Narcissist

How To Neutralize A Narcissist

A Complete Guide on How to Become a Narcissist's Worst Nightmare

Antony Felix

Your Free Gift

As a way of thanking you for the purchase, I'd like to offer you a complimentary gift:

- **5 Pillar Life Transformation Checklist:** This short book is about life transformation, presented in bit size pieces for easy implementation. I believe that without such a checklist, you are likely to have a hard time implementing anything in this book and any other thing you set out to do religiously and sticking to it for the long haul. It doesn't matter whether your goals relate to weight loss, relationships, personal finance, investing, personal development, improving communication in your family, your overall health, finances, improving your sex life, resolving issues in your relationship, fighting PMS successfully, investing, running a successful business, traveling etc. With a checklist like this one, you can bet that anything you do will seem a lot easier to implement until the end. Therefore, even if you don't continue reading this book, at least read the one thing that will help you in every other aspect of your life. Grab your copy now by clicking/tapping here or simply enter http://bit.ly/2fantonfreebie into your browser. Your life will never be the same again (if you implement what's in this book), I promise.

PS: I'd like your feedback. If you are happy with this book, please leave a review on Amazon.

Introduction

Is there someone in your life who constantly seeks validation from you, but fails to show even an ounce of empathy towards you? Do you live with someone who has a grandiose sense of self-image and someone who thinks of everyone as inferior to himself/herself?

Is there someone in your life who showers affection on you when he/she is in need of you, but isn't really there for you when you want his/her comfort? Do you feel you are exploited by a manipulative person in your life who shamelessly takes advantage of you to have a sense of entitlement over you, but does not really care for your feelings?

Do you often suffer from verbal and psychological abuse at the hands of that person who brazenly ridicules and demeans you? Does that very person expect you to appreciate, love and support him/ her all the time without offering you any solace and love in return?

If you answered even a few of these questions with a 'yes', unfortunately you are living with a narcissist who only loves himself/ herself and someone who lacks any sort of compassion for anybody else. A narcissist is someone who suffers from 'Narcissistic Personality Disorder', also known as NPD, which involves arrogant thought process and self-centered behaviors towards others without showing them any consideration, empathy and support while demanding constant attention and validation from them.

A narcissist believes that he/ she is entitled to appreciation, love and admiration from everyone because he/ she is the best and deserves royal treatment. Since he/ she lacks the element of 'empathy' completely, he/ she fails to understand that they also should offer love, care and support to others. Narcissists are often described as manipulative, patronizing, selfish, demanding and extremely cocky. While they can be fun to be around and mostly are very intelligent, living with a narcissist can be more like a never-ending trip to hell.

You may think this is an exaggeration, but this is only the reality. Living with a narcissist can easily take a toll on your body and mind because of their manipulative, controlling and ridiculing behavior towards you. Not only that, but constantly being there for a narcissist and taking care not to ever hurt his/ her feelings can be quite emotionally overwhelming and draining.

Studies show how living with those living with NPD increases your chances of suffering from emotional disorders yourself. While this job is certainly not an easy one, sometimes you just cannot break off with that narcissist in your life. That narcissist may be your sibling, child, friend, colleague, boss, parent, partner or anybody else you share a bond with, or maybe someone you meet occasionally, and even though you are aware of how annoying being around him/ her can be, you know not seeing that person isn't really an option for he/ she isn't really cruel.

What really can one do in that option? The answer is simple: become the narcissist's worst nightmare! It is alright if you do not feel like calling it quits with that person, but you can definitely learn to cope with him/ her effectively without allowing him/her to take charge of your mind. That's right; there is every possibility of you neutralizing the venom of a narcissist so that he/she stops poisoning you, and you too can get some relief.

Are you interested to know how that may happen? This is where this guide serves it purpose. Considering the debilitating and negative influence of narcissists on those living with them and feeling the plight of the sufferers, this guide aims to provide a relief to the latter. It gives you an understanding of NPD, talks about how it can sabotage your life and provides you with potent and actionable information on how to live with a narcissist peacefully without giving him/her the reins to your life. By the time you are done reading this book, you will be invigorated with the power, stamina and motivation to break free of the vicious cycle of manipulation inflicted by narcissists around you and live a happy, confident and meaningful life.

Let's get started.

Table of Contents

Chapter 1: What Living with a Narcissist Looks and Feels Like

Described as having an inflated sense of self-importance, NPD is not just limited to having an interest in your physical appearance. In fact, it is a full-fledged personality disorder that not only damages the victim himself/ herself, but also inflicts irreparable damage on to the ones living with him/ her.

Sneak Peak into Narcissism

Psychologist Stephen Johnson aptly describes a narcissist as someone who has buried his/ her genuine self-expression due to different traumatic experiences he/she suffered in life and replaced that with a compensatory and highly developed false self. The compensatory false sense of self that narcissists form makes them somehow cope with problems in life, but turns them into egotistical and conceited individuals. One does feel like empathizing with a narcissist at times, but mostly, narcissist wreak such a havoc in the lives of others that it becomes quite impossible to even understand their viewpoint.

Narcissism basically stems from a lack of genuine self-worth, which is primarily due to the unavailability of emotional support and nourishment in the childhood or adolescence years.

So yes, nobody is born a narcissist, but is made one. Since they fail to receive the care, emotional support and attention they yearn for in life, they do not have a high, genuine sense of self-esteem. To cope with this dearth of self-belief and confidence, narcissists create an outer shell of ego and a grandiose sense of self-worth to cope with the pain they once suffered.

While the narcissists' coping mechanism may be rooted in their honest and innocent intention, it soon takes off an ugly, twisted turn when they cannot see beyond themselves. This then makes things difficult for those living with them, working with them or sharing a relationship with them in any capacity. If you worry you are living with a narcissist or know of someone who shows signs of being a narcissist, you can relate to this pain.

The good news is you can learn ways to cope with them and neutralize their dominating effect, but for that, you must first be sure whether or not you are living with a narcissist.

Let us take a look at how living with a narcissist feels like and the signs that a loved one is a narcissist.

Signs That You Have a Narcissist Around You

A narcissist is certain that he/ she alone deserves to be treated with utmost respect and love, and nobody else is worthy of that attention. This attitude along with many of their behaviors can make you feel throttled.

Let me explain that:

1: You are treated like an object by them

Narcissists believe that they have complete entitlement over people they share a close bond with due to which they feel all their demands must met. They are likely to approach you for favors and requests every now and then, many of which feel like demands and orders instead of request.

For instance, if they want you to help them out with a project, they won't politely ask you to do it, but would just pass an order. This behavior makes you feel like an object or their slave who must only do as they want.

If you feel that a certain loved one, friend or person in your life makes you feel that their needs are far greater and important than yours, and shows a complete disregard to your feelings and needs, you are living with a narcissist and the feeling is not a nice one.

2: You are threatened by them

If there is someone in your life who frequently threatens to leave you, expose any of your shortcomings or a mistake you are not too proud of, or harm you in any way when you do not do as they command, it is likely he/ she is a narcissist.

For example, being told by your friend that he/ she will tell your partner about your affair with your classmate before your marriage; or being threatened by your partner that he/ she will leave you if you do not support them financially are examples of being threatened by a narcissist.

Since narcissists believe they are entitled to treat you in whatever way they like, if you ever choose to disagree with them, you will only trigger their volatile behavior, which may involve the use of threats and abusive behavior.

3: *You are trapped into guilt by them*

Narcissists have a habit of making one feel guilty and at fault all the time. If you are made to feel that whatever you do is because the goodwill/help of the narcissist in your life, that they are the reason you have gotten far ahead in life and that you cannot succeed on your own, you are living with a narcissist. Moreover, if something wrong happens to them, then too, you are blamed for it and made to feel guilty. Statements like 'I am the reason you are earning well', 'I am the one who encouraged you to pursue your dreams', 'You could never do this on your own', 'See, things go wrong when you don't listen to me' and the likes are often hurled at you by a narcissist.

Narcissists are also master manipulators who constantly attempt to make you feel discouraged and guilty whenever they get the chance. All of this can feel very draining and can often make you cry for mercy. If you feel that way, it is clear you are living with a narcissist.

4: They Expect Grand Treatment from You

The minute the narcissist in your life walks in the house or meets you, he/ she is likely to want the best treatment from you. He/ she may want you to talk to him/ her with utmost respect, not go against their wishes and even seek their permission before doing anything with your own life. If your partner or a loved one forces you to treat him/ her like a messiah, does not observe any rules himself/ herself, and forces others to behave impeccably while he/ she may not do the same himself/ herself, your life is likely to be a very tough one. It is not easy running around on your toes doing one thing after another just to please that person.

Moreover, despite all your efforts, that person is still likely to be displeased with you at the end of the day. Complains by your addict mother that you are never there for her; or by your partner that you never really loved him/her are classic examples of how the narcissists are never pleased with you and keep increasing their demands.

5: They Play Games with You and Subject You to Gaslighting

Narcissists go through a lot of mood swings and temperament issues. Their attitude and behavior keeps shifting from hot to cold time and again. While they are mostly demanding, they can become incredibly sweet, caring and loving when they want something from you, and sense you may get assertive or leave them if they act dominating.

The moment they become sweet, you are likely to melt down for them and agree to their whims. While you may believe they have changed for the better and things will finally be fine, you realize how wrong you were when you see them changing colors soon after and returning to their old, cold, controlling demeanor. This keeps going on and on, and is likely to make you go crazy.

It is a normal, natural demand to want stability in life, but life with a narcissist can never get stable because their games never stop. When you do confront them about their behavior, they are likely to gaslight you and blame it all on you. In their defense, they will argue that you made them do whatever it is they did; that their actions were as a result of your actions. To them, there can only be something wrong; your narcissist partner or loved one or acquaintance believes he/she can never be wrong.

6: Can Be Very Competitive

There are two broad categories of narcissists: vulnerable and grandiose narcissists.

The former has an outward exterior of self-absorption and self-centeredness with a very weak inner core. Such people demand appreciation and validation from others because they hardly have any accomplishment to themselves which makes them feel inferior to others.

The second type, the grandiose narcissists, on the other hand, truly believe in their abilities and greatness, and are likely to be as good as they feel they are. Both the types have their own problems and both types display the signs discussed before. That said, with the grandiose narcissists comes another problem: extreme competition. If someone is a grandiose narcissist, for instance, he/ she is likely to give you a very hard time progressing at work. He/ she will want all the promotions, incentives and bonuses for him/herself, and may even resort to mean games and conspiracies if he/she feels you are a competition for him/ her. This can make enjoying your work and excelling in it very tough for you.

This issue can also prevail if you have a partner, a friend or a sibling who is a grandiose narcissist. He/ she is likely to compare his/her work, promotions, career opportunities, financial success and growth with you, and if he/ she is doing better than you, it is likely he/ she will rub it in your face time and again making you feel inferior. In case you are doing better, he/ she is likely to turn bitter towards you and this is likely to reflect in his/ her weird, irrational behavior.

7: There are No Limits to the Extent a Narcissist Can Go to

A narcissist rarely has any sense of proportion which means that anything can ignite their volatile temper, and when he/ she gets really angry, you cannot gauge the limit to which he/ she could go to because there is no limit.

Narcissists struggle with determining the varying levels of different problems and reacting/ responding accordingly. The pettiest of issues can set him/ her off and make them behave irrationally with you.

So whether you forgot to put enough salt in the rice, or didn't iron the right shirt your partner asked you, it can easily trigger him off and make him resort to even violent behavior with you. A life with such uncertainty and one where you never know what may upset the other person is certainly quite a chaotic one. It takes a toll on your body and mind, and can easily deplete your self-confidence, positivity and sanity.

How can you remain and act sanely if you are always living in a volcano? While this is hard and there may be times when you just want to cut off from the person completely, you cannot always do that for different reasons. Sometimes, that narcissist may just be a colleague whom you have to see at work, and you cannot leave your job that you're passionate about just because of him/her. And other times, even though the narcissist may be your partner, you may know you love him/ her too much to break up with him/her.

Whatever your reasons are for staying with the narcissist for the long haul, there is a possibility of things working out for you two. However, for that to happen, you need to gear up and work on yourself to build a personality that deflects their strikes every time and keeps you sane enough even amidst the mayhem. The following chapters of the book will guide you on how to do that so you can transform yourself into a narcissist's worst nightmare so every time a narcissist thinks of manipulating you, he/ she thinks thrice.

Chapter 2: Maintain a Positive Outlook in Life and Calm Yourself Down

Dealing with a narcissist is not easy but it is nonetheless possible. To take up on this huge challenge and accomplish it, you need your sanity first. If you are emotionally drained, weak and unhappy, you will not be able to face him/ her, combat your troubles and deflect the criticism, abuse and trauma he/ she inflicts on you in any way. You need to befriend yourself first, become your most important ally and change your outlook towards life so you start living optimistically and can handle that egoistic control freak in your life appropriately.

Your Sanity Comes First

If you are emotionally unstable and depressed, you won't be able to tackle the challenge that lies ahead of you. You will forever feel terrible from within and allow the misery to take over you completely. This has to change. This must change for only then will you equip yourself with the courage, resilience, strength and optimism you need to handle that narcissist in your life and move forward happily.

For you to feel sane and happy, there are a few changes you need to bring to your mindset and beliefs. Our beliefs, however they are, shape our entire life including our behavior, feelings and attitude. If you think you cannot be happy, you will become unhappy and live an unhappy life. However, if you choose to believe that you have every right to being happy, you will *choose* to be happy no matter what.

In an ideal condition, every athlete running a marathon has an equal chance of making it to the finish line. However, some do not make it to the finish line. The difference between those who achieve victory and those who don't isn't always in their capabilities, but more in their mindset. You may think you cannot survive this life at all and that no matter what, you will stay miserable. Trust me, if you strongly believe that, this is what will happen; your beliefs shape your internal program created by your subconscious mind.

When you constantly focus on a certain thought, emotion, feeling or suggestion, it is picked up by the Reticular Activating System (RAS) in your brain as something important to you. This very system is in charge of filtering out irrelevant pieces of information from your memory to prevent information overload. It does keep whatever you focus on or repeat the most because that is how it interprets the significance of different things for you. Hence, when you focus on something, think about it time and again, and become emotionally invested in it, it is perceived as important for you. It then becomes a part of your belief system and influences you in every aspect. Thinking that you can never be happy, live confidently or progress while you are with your narcissist; or feeling that there is no hope for you are unhealthy beliefs, which then shape your life accordingly. A major reason why you haven't been able to handle your narcissist effectively is your unhealthy beliefs.

For you to move towards a happy life, one where you feel in charge of yourself and your life, and can make your own decisions, you need to change your beliefs for the better. Here are some beliefs you should work on to build a healthier, happier mindset.

Make a Decision

First and foremost, you need to make a clear decision on how you wish to live your life. Think of how the one or more narcissists in your life are treating you, and if it is not a pleasant feeling and makes you feel suffocated, hurt and ridiculed, make a decision to turn things around. Think of all the things you have ever wanted to do in life and write them down in your journal.

Next, think of all the ways the narcissists in your life are sabotaging your wellbeing and keep you from becoming better. Write down how you feel and think of the positive improvements you will be able to bring in your life once you block out their hazardous effects. Think of how you will feel good about yourself; how you will finally have some time and sanity to focus on your wellbeing and needs; how you will stop taking orders from them and do things as you want; how you will stop being their caregiver 24/7 and look after yourself for a change too; how you will stop worrying about pleasing them; and how you will finally focus on your growth, happiness and success.

Make a mental picture of these things and reflect on how happy that would make you. This is what you aim and deserve to achieve, and you can have all that and more by just moving from the passenger seat of your life's car to its driving seat. It is best to write this decision down on paper in order to commit yourself to it for real and solidify your commitment. Next, start taking baby steps towards this goal by working on building some healthy beliefs.

Change the Victim Mentality

The very first belief that you need to improve on is the victim mentality you have nurtured for a long time. While living with or being in any sort of relationship with a controlling narcissist especially one with a grandiose sense of self-worth can make you feel like the victim, this is not the reality. The truth is *that the narcissist is really the person with a problematic mindset.* It is him/ her whose behavior and thought process isn't proper. He/ she may not feel like the victim, but he/ she is the patient and has turned you into a miserable person too

That said, you still have the sanity to see through things and think rationality, and that is a blessing in itself. You may feel like the victim, but you are not and you can easily turn the tables in your favor if you stop acting like the victim. Narcissists have the habit to control and boss around people. Whether it is your narcissist neighbor who keeps asking you for favors and makes you feel you are obliged to pay heed to him; or it is your narcissistic elder sister who loves dominating you, that person knows how to pull your strings and that's what he/ she has been doing for a long while. This is exactly why you feel like a victim and keep giving in to his/ her whims and wishes. But, this has to change and it can only change if you become the real boss of your life.

Here is what you should do.

- Give Yourself Positive Suggestions: Every time you feel you are a victim and are just being viciously pulled in the manipulation cycle of a narcissist, remind yourself of your goal. Think of the commitment you made to yourself and use that to change your victim mindset. Tell yourself out loud 'I am the real boss of my life and I live on my terms' instead of saying 'I am not a victim.' When you repeat suggestions with words such as 'no', 'not' or 'never' in them, they aren't received well by your subconscious. Your mind does not accept words with negative connotations so when you tell yourself not to do something, it does exactly that as the 'not' gets omitted from the suggestion. If you remind yourself of how you are *not* the victim, it will, one way or another, make you feel like the actual victim. The right way is to remind yourself of how you are the *boss* and must act like one. Soon, you will find yourself becoming emotionally strong to do just as you want.

- Start Making Small Decisions for Yourself: Telling yourself that you rule your life won't only work, you need to prove that too. No need to panic and jump on to big decisions instantly; just start small and keep building the way up. Start off with things like deciding what to wear, the meals to cook, what grocery to do and the likes. If you feel like wearing blue and putting on some makeup (for women), do it. If you wish to dine out alone, go do it. Take very small, baby steps and even that will be enough for now to prove you how you are capable of deciding things for yourself.

- Be Firm: When you make even the littlest of decisions, the narcissist in your life, especially if you live with him/ her, will try to throttle you. Your narcissistic colleague won't like if you are the team lead and ask your team to work in a certain manner. Neither will your narcissist spouse approve of you decorating your bedroom a certain way, but you need to stick to what you do. If the little decisions that you take do not affect his/ her health and life in any negative way, there is no reason to feel bad about your decision. Just firmly tell him/ her that you like things a certain way or wish to do something and you will do it. Yes, standing up to him/ her for your right will be hard, and may overwhelm you at first, but if you stay resolved, he/ she won't be able to break you. As much as narcissists love to dominate and portray themselves as super-strong individuals, they aren't as strong from within and if you come off as the stronger and more assertive person, you are likely to shake them up a bit which will make them back off.

- Remind Yourself of Your Needs and Goals: Every time you feel unconfident about moving forward, remind yourself of what you aspire to do in life and how much your own body and mind need your very attention. Think of these things, take out your journal and go through the commitment you wrote on it some time back to refuel your motivation to keep moving forward and become the boss of your life.

Remember that implementing these techniques once or twice won't do the trick; you have to work on them consistently to nurture the habit of thinking positively at all times.

Life is Good

If you are unhappy in your life and not pleased with the way the narcissists treat you, you are likely to believe how your life is unfair and not good. This is justified, to some extent, but if you recall what we wrote above on how what you repeatedly tell yourself turns into your belief, you will realize that your life feels miserable also because you keep telling yourself how it is like that. Hardships are an inevitable part of everyone's life, but your approach and outlook towards life is what determines how and what you will manifest.

You need to stop telling yourself of how bad your life is and focus on the good parts.

Every day, think of any 3 things to be thankful for. Put your house, warm food, clean clothes, the ability to breathe etc. on the list every single day and pay your gratitude for all these blessings. Think of how there are people living with even far less and stuck in more unfortunate conditions, and how you have the chance to change your life for the better. Do that and tell yourself of how you are responsible of manifesting the reality of your life. You do this persistently; you will actually feel confident to take a stand for yourself.

You Have Every Right to Be Happy

Never tell yourself of how you cannot be happy, or just because you chose to be with the wrong person in case your spouse is a narcissist, you deserve to be treated badly. Nobody deserves to be unhappy or treated poorly, and if someone is inflicting any sort of pain or abuse on another person, the abused must stand for their rights.

Whenever you feel upset, controlled and overlooked by the narcissist, remind yourself of how you deserve to be happy. Moreover, chant this affirmation 'I am happy and deserve to be happy' several times clearly, loudly and confidently throughout the day. An affirmation is anything you believe to be true which mostly happens when you repeat something time and again. When you recurrently chant 'I am happy', you will activate your RAS, which will them embrace that suggestion and soon imbed it in your subconscious. Soon enough, you will start to feel happy from within which will encourage you more to look after your wellbeing.

You Can Do it

Another belief that you need to work on is that you can do anything you want. Narcissists can often deplete your confidence due to gaslighting, emotional abuse and the constant act of blaming you for every problem. This is likely to make you feel that you are incapable of achieving anything in life. If you wish to break this cycle, want to progress in your career, want to be happy and want to live a well-balanced life, you need to build a can-do attitude.

Chant suggestions like 'I am working on my goals and fulfilling them' and 'I am living for myself and making progress with each passing day' at least 20 times throughout the day so that you slowly transform yourself into a doer from a complainer.

While consistently working on these tips, also practice different strategies to stay composed and strong throughout the process because that helps you keep your emotions in check and deal the narcissists around you effectively. The next chapter throws more light on this.

Chapter 3: Relax, Compose Yourself and Become Mindful of Yourself

Staying composed and poised throughout this time is crucial to your wellbeing. Also, you will only be able to control the narcissists around you effectively if you stay calm and composed.

If you lose your temper or keep getting agitated by their irrational behavior, you won't be able to stick to your mission and may give in to their manipulation. Also, you need to learn to keep your emotions in check so you do not exhibit your agitation to the narcissist.

Narcissists love playing with one's emotions and feelings. When they sense they can get under your skin, they are likely to try manipulating you even more which will only upset you and strain your bond with him/ her. It is important to become more aware of how you feel and the different things that trigger your annoyance so you can manage those triggers and keep yourself calm. When you stay calm, you are better able to handle the narcissists around you too.

When you are calm, you are likely not to react to their demeaning behavior, which will only piss them off and make them explode. Not only that, but your reaction, be it volatile or surrendering to their whims is what they yearn for. Narcissists feed on your misery so if you keep feeling miserable, they only grow more powerful.

To become their nightmare, you need to stop allowing them to get the better of you. Reacting to their behavior needs to stop and must be replaced with 'responding.' Responding to something means you analyze the situation before reacting to it impulsively so you think things through and make an informed decision.

To tactfully handle a narcissist, you need to be equipped with these powerful skills, which you can develop through mindfulness. Let's discuss how mindfulness can help you to control/tame a narcissist and neutralize their venom.

How Mindfulness Helps You Control Narcissists and Neutralize their Venom

Mindfulness refers to living in the moment peacefully, acceptingly and nonjudgmentally. Narcissists can be extremely controlling and this can easily make you nurture a pessimistic attitude towards life. You either worry about what may happen next, or rehash all the painful memories. Either way, you ignore the present you live in and keep burdening yourself with more worries. To overpower the narcissists you have to deal with, you need to be stronger and more conscious of how you feel, and this can only happen if you live in the moment.

If you are forgetful (opposite of being mindful), you are likely not to pay attention to how the narcissist in your life controls you and won't come up with appropriate strategies to deflect their strikes. For instance, you may not realize that every time your partner sees you feeling upset after he/ she has thrown an irrational tantrum, he/ she soon comes up with a sweet apology to cheer you up, and you give in to his/ her tactics every single time.

You allow the narcissists in your life to play with your feeling which is why you are never able to really step up your game. Also, the inability to live in the moment is what makes you react to their tantrums instead of just blocking their moves and exiting the volatile situation. If your seemingly best friend shouts at you and makes a mountain out of molehill of every petty issue each time things don't go his/ her way, you need to stop reacting to it by explaining yourself every time.

Instead, you just need to stay quiet, acknowledge that he/ she is again having a meltdown, which you cannot do anything about and simply leave. While you may think the second approach won't affect them, this is what will break them from within. When they see you not reacting to their moves and simply keep your emotions intact, they will slowly break from within.

Not only that, but mindfulness also instills in you calmness and peacefulness, which you need to keep your sanity in check and stay poised at all times so you stay optimistic and focus on yourself more than the narcissist. Arguably, the best way to inculcate mindfulness is to practice meditation.

Why Meditate

Meditation is a practice that can instill in you mindfulness and the ability to live in the moment peacefully and nonjudgmentally. It does so by relaxing your chaotic state of mind, calms your racing thoughts and helps you focus better by giving you some break between the scores of thoughts running haphazardly in your head.

When you are able to let go of this frenzy, you get more time in between thoughts and this can greatly help you to relax, focus better and also become more mindful. Meditation achieves this by regulating your brainwaves and by slowly training you to bring your attention to the moment you experience.

In addition, meditation can help you to enjoy the following positive results:

- Unlock your creativity

- Think deeply

- Become more intuitive

- Develop a positive attitude and can-do mindset

- Strengthen relationships

- Think rationally

- Boost overall cognition and memory

- Improve heart health

- Reduce chances of developing diabetes and high blood pressure

- Improve overall health and help cope with arthritis, digestive issues and back pains

- Boost your immunity

- Combat stress, anxiety and depression which you are likely to experience frequently while living with a narcissist

- Build better control over your emotions so you stop surrendering to the never ending demands of narcissists

Obviously, the above are not all the benefits; everyone is likely to notice some unique benefits that the other person may not experience. Since that's not the main focus of this book, let's move on to something else. Let me share a powerful meditation technique that you can use to keep yourself calm, confident, happy and manage narcissists effectively.

Mindfulness Meditation

This simple meditation technique requires you to focus better on the moment while using your breath as the object of your focus. You align your attention with your breath and observe it throughout the meditation session. The first few sessions are likely to be difficult, as you will find yourself struggling to maintain focus even for a few minutes, but if you keep at it, you only improve with time.

The next few sessions will leave you feeling peaceful and happy from within. You will feel more relaxed and focused on the moment, and will begin to understand what staying in the moment actually means. This will slowly help you bring your attention to the moment every time it wanders off in thought and you will enjoy your normal everyday tasks more instead of doing them casually while only worrying about the narcissistic abuse you experience.

After a month or two of meditating, you will find yourself feeling more in control of your thoughts and the emotions they bring about in you. You will also stop allowing the narcissists around you to control you by listening to their demands and obeying them round the clock. Instead, you will focus more on what you want, stand up for yourself and stop acting like their doormat. With that in mind, let's discuss how you can accomplish that.

Find a nice, peaceful spot to meditate in and sit comfortably in any pose you like. Cross your legs or spread them in front of you, or lie down on the bed or sit in a chair. Next, start becoming more mindful of your breath by slowly becoming attentive of it.

Whatever it is that you were thinking earlier on, let go of it and simply observe your breath. Breathe through your nose when you inhale and expel the air out through your mouth. There is no need to deepen the breath now; just breathe naturally while focusing on your breath. Observing your breath means you watch it as it enters your body, circulates inside, produces certain sensations and then moves out of your system. Therefore, when you inhale and exhale, just watch your breath and use that as an anchor to become grounded to the moment.

You may find your thoughts wandering off and on, and this is quite natural and normal at this point. Just stay calm and count your breath if you need to every time you feel distracted. Gently bring back your attention to your breath and the present moment, and you will feel much better shortly.

Carry out this practice for a good 5 minutes and you will be amazed at how serene you soon feel from within. Ensure to do it at least once daily especially when you feel extremely confused and with time, do it more frequently. The more you practice it, the better you become at it and the more you stay mindful of your thoughts and feelings. With time, this very practice will make you realize how futile it is to react to the different manipulative tactics used by narcissists and focus more on your wellbeing. Additionally, you will be able to better reflect on your thoughts, aspirations and desires and figure out better what you want in life. This will give you a clearer direction and purpose, which you can follow to add meaning to your life.

It is not just the narcissists in your life who enjoy controlling you, but in some way, you too have become used to this manipulation, which often makes you feel as if taking care of them is your sole purpose in life. You cannot focus on yourself and neutralize their negativity unless you have a clear and strong motivation in your life.

When you discover yourself better, you move closer to understanding your purpose in life, and once you dig that out, you know what you are supposed to do in life. This realization alone is enough to compel you to shield yourself from the narcissists and become even stronger than them.

Respond and Not React to the Tactics

With the passage of time, you will find yourself feeling more poised and mindful. This will help you inculcate the ability to stay firm and strong when the narcissist around you tries to pick up a fight with you, force you to do as he/ she wants and ridicules you. There is no need to react to their manipulative behavior because that's how they get under your skin. They know they can pull your strings like a puppet easily by sometime being sweet, angry, controlling and comforting.

If you are upset with your partner and decide to act assertively, he/she is likely to remind you of everything he/she ever did to make you happy. If that won't work, he/she may then play the blame game and tell you how you ruined his/her life. If that does not work its magic like it used to, he/she is likely to act apologetically. He/she will keep trying different moves to break you such that you let go of your decision and continue to live with him/her on his/her terms. In this situation, you need to make sure you do not react to anything he/she says and silently focus on your own thing.

To do that, make sure to do the following:

- Keep practicing meditation regularly so that you have more control of your thoughts.

- Every time you sense a narcissist around you taking advantage of you or talking rudely to you, or doing anything you do not like, simply move away from the situation.

- Do not shout or say anything negative when the narcissist misbehaves for a few times; observe his/ her behavior to get to the root of the problem. If this continues, you will have to take a stand for yourself which I will teach you how in the chapters to follow.

- Take deep breaths when you sense anger building up inside you to calm yourself down and think rationally.

Work on these tactics to stay composed and choose the high road every time a narcissist misbehaves. At the same time, try to dig deeper in the problem by understanding where their irrational behavior comes from.

Evaluate the Context and Figure Out where Their Behavior Comes From

The awareness and mindfulness you inculcate in yourself will come in handy when you want to better understand the narcissists you wish to handle better. You need to slowly become assertive with them without acting negatively or resorting to negative measures like they do.

Always remember that narcissists, especially the vulnerable kind, need someone to make them feel better about themselves. This is why they start undercutting and sneaking. When you become assertive, they are likely to question your power to create more mischief. If you understand that they are mainly coming from a place of intense insecurity and not just dominance, you can then offer them with enough reassurance that settles them down so you focus on what needs to be done.

You need to be very careful when reassuring them as an overabundance of it will only fan their ego, but when done right, it will calm them down and also help you slowly take control over them. So if you see your narcissistic friend asking you on how he/ she looks, you compliment him/ her nicely. However, if your narcissistic partner forces you to leave your job when you clearly don't want to, you put your foot down and explain to him how you won't succumb to their demand, but also remind them of how much you love him/her and expect him/her to understand your passion. You soon learn to manipulate the narcissists as well without leaving your stance or feeling confused.

You also need to evaluate the context of the situation that makes a narcissist react and behave a certain way. Narcissism is an all-or-nothing character trait, which means that the narcissist will either be good or bad. They see in only black or white, and can never understand the grey areas.

To handle them effectively, you need to understand their personality trait. For instance, if a colleague was turned down for a promotion he was eagerly anticipating, and now has to work with you because you received the promotion, you will have to understand why he has become spiteful and vindictive with you. If you just evaluate the context of the situation that unleashed the monster inside him/her, you are likely to behave accordingly with him/her instead of losing your temper.

As you slowly start to cope with them better in a more thoughtful and accepting manner without reassuring them more than they need, you need to slowly prove to them that you can manage things on your own and are capable of becoming independent and strong in all aspects. The next chapter will teach you how to achieve that.

Chapter 4: Value Yourself and Show Them You Can Manage Alone (Financially Emotionally etc)

The ulterior motive (even if they cannot publicly acknowledge it) of every narcissist is to make those who bear with their behavior more dependent on them so that every time a person tries to make a decision, he/ she seeks the support of the narcissist to do it. It is likely the narcissist you are dealing with, whether it is your boss, friend, sibling or partner tries his/ her best to cripple your ability to act independently so that you rely entirely on him/ her. For everything that you wish to do in life, you will have to seek his/ her permission and this only damages your self-esteem, confidence and wellbeing in general.

You need to show him/ her that you can function alone, in fact, show him/her that you are very happy on your own and do not need his/ her shoulder for support every time. This does not mean you leave him/ her; it means you should try to prove to him/ her that you are capable of managing things on your own. For that, you need to start valuing yourself and look after yourself.

Here is how you can go about this goal.

Take Care of Your Health

Make a start by paying better attention to your health. The old age adage 'health is wealth' holds truth because without good health, you can never achieve any goal in life. To combat the manipulative power of a narcissist, you need to think straight which cannot happen if you feel weak or are always too lethargic to do anything.

Lethargy and weakness are both caused by unhealthy diet and unhealthy habits. Therefore, Pay attention to your health and focus on the different health issues you are facing, if any. In case you feel unwell or suffer from body pains or any other ailment, get it diagnosed and then observe its treatment procedure strictly. Meanwhile, bring healthy changes to your diet by eating wholesome, fresh foods that provide you with a good dose of good fats, protein, carbohydrates, minerals, vitamins, fiber and water. Eat healthy and stay hydrated while indulging in some guilty pleasures like your favorite double cheese pizza or the fudge cake you often crave for every once in a while.

Moreover, make sure not to starve yourself at any cost and space your meals with 2 to 3 hours in between. If you struggle with managing your weight, it is quite likely the narcissists in your life body shame you often to manipulate you. This can easily intimidate and upset you making you resort to extreme measures to lose or gain weight which will affect your wellbeing and sanity. Here is an example to help you understand what I mean by this.

Leslie, 36 lived with a narcissist partner who used to body shame her every now and then, something which only made her feel bad about herself. Since she weighed around 200 pounds whereas her partner had a more athletic body, Leslie felt indebted to him for living with her and allowed him to manipulate and control her for that very reason. However, with the help of some trustworthy friends, she realized how her partner was abusing her and slowly gained self-confidence to show him that she too can live on her own without him. When Leslie gained more confidence, she was soon able to intimidate her partner and control him without allowing him to damage her self-esteem.

You too can achieve that state of mind and be able to have control over the narcissists in your life by making a start with looking after your health. Eat healthy, take your medicines if you have to and listen to what your body wants.

Sleep Well

You need to sleep well, as much as you need, because that too affects your wellbeing and sanity. A good night's sleep, as research shows ,can help you think clearly, feel happy, act confidently and stay mindful without giving in to the clever tactics of the narcissists around you. Research also shows that adults need 7 to 9 hours of sleep on average to act rationally, feel good and take control of yourself. If you are getting less sleep than that, it is time to sleep better because it is only when you feel relaxed that you will be able to thwart the moves of narcissists effectively.

To do that, do the following:

- Set specific sleep and wake up times, and stick to them. If you intend to sleep at 11am, do so no matter what even if your partner wants to talk to you at that very hour. Similarly, wake up at 7am if that's your plan, even if you keep tossing and turning at night. If you stick to these times over a period of a few weeks, your body will soon adjust to the new routine and adhere to it.

- Unwind an hour before your sleep time by doing something relaxing such as taking a warm bath or reading a soothing book so you can relax and sleep easily.

- Make sure your bedspread, pillow and mattress are comfortable to sleep on so you relax and can initiate sleep easily when you are on your bed.

- Meditate for a few minutes before sleeping in order to relax and fall asleep easily without focusing on distracting thoughts.

Work on these guidelines over a period of a few weeks and soon, you will find yourself sleeping well. This will help you feel healthy, happy and confident so you focus on yourself and not on the control freaks in your life.

Stay Active

Staying active is crucial to a healthy and happy life, and if you live a sedentary life, that also explains why you feel lethargic, unhappy and cannot focus well on your wellbeing. Also, when a narcissist sees you moving actively and doing everything energetically, he/ she will get the clear message that you are capable of acting independently and can function without his/ her support.

Start doing things on your own instead of always asking someone to do them for you. If you want a plate from the kitchen, get up and grab it. Also, slowly incorporate at least 10 minutes of physical activity in your routine to boost the production of mood improving hormones in your body such as serotonin and dopamine that boost your mood and confidence. You could play a sport, dance, do Pilates, do kickboxing or any other activity you enjoy.

With time, you will feel more energetic, have increased stamina and will also feel more positive to effectively look after yourself and block the negativity spewed on you by the narcissistic, manipulative person in your life.

Understand and Address Your Physical, Emotional and Spiritual Needs

While you do the above, pay attention to your other physical, emotional, spiritual and any other needs you may have to feel good and confident about yourself.

If you need to get new clothes or shoes, invest some money in yourself. Maybe, get a nice haircut or visit the spa. You may also wish to be around someone who understands your misery, feels your pain and supports you in return. Seek such company by reaching out to supportive family and friends, looking up support groups online and attend different meet-ups and events that suit your interests. If there is a book club that holds regular sessions and you love reading, attend a session and make new friends.

You need to constantly be watching your needs and taking care to fulfill them on time. You have not done that in a long while which is another reason why you feel like a victim and have allowed narcissists around you to rule you. Remember, the world only respects those who respect themselves, and that can only happen when you look after your wellbeing.

Build Skills

Confidence is the key character trait you need to build to stand up against narcissists around you and become unattractive for them. Self-confidence is rooted in your self-esteem, which comes from different things among which is your skill set.

If you are talented and have a skill or an entire skill set to boast about, you will automatically feel good about yourself. You know you are capable of doing things, something which makes you value yourself. As a result, your confidence levels are likely to be high.

Narcissists have a habit of downplaying other people's feelings by reminding them of how incompetent they are. If you can prove them wrong by doing something really well or proving your talent by developing a skill or two, you will instantly knock them down.

Find out what you are good at, capable of doing and feel inclined to pursue and build a skill focusing on that area. If you love to paint, maybe take proper, professional painting classes and then pursue it as a profession. If you enjoy robotics and artificial intelligence, you could learn to build robots from online tutorials, or enroll into a proper program if you can. Focus on constantly improving your skill set in order to get better with time. You can then try your luck in different areas and achieve more in life.

Also, remember to become the best in the one area you are good at. If coding is your thing, constantly push yourself to be better than ever. This ups your game, opens up new opportunities for you and makes you strive for excellence. When the narcissist around you sees you constantly excelling in life, they only feel miserable from within. Also, when they see you growing more confident and emotionally strong, they find it difficult to manipulate you.

Move Forward in Professional Life

If you do not have a career yet, focus on having one now even if you are not too motivated to have a professional life. You are on a mission to neutralize the effect of narcissists around you and show them that you can function independently. To make this possible, becoming financially independent is crucial.

One way or another, you know you have a backup in the form of that narcissist in your life to love, support and care for you even though their care and love is superficial. If that person is responsible for your financial sustenance, you are quite likely not to focus on it yourself and rely on him/ her.

However, things have to change now; you are not the same person as you were before i.e. one who would keep up with abuse inflicted on him/ her. You have to prove the narcissists around you wrong. They think you cannot do it without them, but you can. As you build a certain skill, start to offer that as a service or product to people through freelancing sites, social media groups and other channels. For instance, if you enjoy making candles, you can turn your passion into a business and sell candles. Make a business page of it on social media platforms and even a website for it if possible. Even if you earn a mere $20 from it in the start, you will feel more confident of yourself because it shows how you can do things on your own.

Keep moving forward steadily by investing more time, effort and money in your business to grow it bigger and become more successful with time. If, however, you are interested in doing some job, look for some relevant to your expertise, skills and prior experience, if any. Once you land a nice job, put in your best effort in it and keep seeking different opportunities to excel in your career.

Whatever money you earn from your profession, save at least 50% of it, especially if the narcissist you are trying to control is your partner and is responsible for providing you with financial assistance. If the two of you are living together, it is his/her right to contribute to the household expenses, and if he/she does that, do not refuse to take money. However, if he/ she objects to your profession and forces you to leave it, tell him/ her firmly that in that case, you will only separate from him and will keep your job. He/she is quite dependent on you, and is likely to budge from his/ her stance when he/ she sees you stick to yours.

Improve Your Financial Life

Keep working hard to increase your income and climb up the success ladder professionally as this helps improve your financial life as well as your self-confidence. Confidence is rooted in your accomplishments, and being able to earn for yourself or your family is a huge confidence booster and accomplishment. Hence, keep working hard to earn more and crush the narcissists around you from within. Also, if you have narcissistic colleagues, moving up the success ladder will only shatter their superficial sense of self-worth and slowly cripple their ability to ridicule and control you.

Let me give you an example.

Jason, 26 recalls living with a narcissistic roommate in college 3 years ago. The roommate used to lend Jason money to help him pay his tuition fee and slowly used that as the reason to manipulate and control him. Jason remembers how he used to live more like his friend's slave and had no life of his own. With the help of his girlfriend who chose to stick to him despite his lack of control on his own life, he soon realized the narcissistic abuse he was suffering from. Without informing his friend, he started looking for jobs and soon found one. Within 6 months, he was able to make a decent amount of money and one fine day, after 2 years of struggle, he paid back his friend all the debt. He felt free and then firmly told his narcissistic friend how he would not surrender to his wishes then. Jason remembers how startled his friend looked and slowly withdrew his controlling behavior.

Make Decisions on Your Own

As your confidence levels slowly perk up, you will feel more in control of your life and will find in you the courage to take decisions for yourself. Continuing with Jason's example, he also shares how he found the courage to make decisions for himself as his financial life and confidence levels perked up. Now that he knew he was doing things for himself, he did not feel obliged to his friend to do things his way and started taking decisions on his own. This again was a massive confidence booster for him as he slowly felt more in control of his life.

You too need to do the same to feel that your life belongs to you only. From deciding what to wear to what activities to take part in to which friends to hang out with to how to invest your money to everything else- take shots yourself instead of looking up to the different authority figures in your life.

As you slowly bring these positive improvements in your life, your narcissistic colleagues, partner, friends and siblings will only feel more intimidated by you. They will realize how independent, strong and capable you are, and while they may not agree to it up front, deep down, they will accept your capabilities. This will discourage them from dictating/controlling you and will slowly start to act submissively towards you.

The truth however is that not all narcissists will break down by this, but they will definitely stop taking you over.

Take Responsibility Of Your Decisions

Not every decision that you make will turn out to be favorable for you. You are a human who is bound to err so you too will have slip-ups and make bad decisions. During such times, keep your calm and do not feel demotivated. Your narcissistic partner or friend, however, will use that as an opportunity to make you feel bad and may even ridicule you. You need to maintain your calm and take responsibility of your decisions.

Instead of telling them how much you regret trying to do things on your own, apologizing to them for not listening to them and promising them to do as they say because they have your best interests at heart, prove them wrong by taking full responsibility of your life and decisions. Accept your mistakes, but also tell them that the slip-ups helped you grow and that you do not regret taking them. If and when they demean you or make fun of you, firmly tell them to behave nicely with you and leave. Instead of reacting to their nonsensical behavior, take the high road and do not say anything and just smile at their ignorance.

Just keep working on these tactics and soon enough, you will feel content, happy and assured from within. The narcissists around you will also realize your might and will slowly stop bothering you because they now know how you aren't weak anymore and will leave them if they continue to try to overshadow and control you.

You also need to set some clear boundaries in your relationship with the different narcissists in your life, learn to be assertive when the need arises and tweak your behavior around them so they know you will not take any of their abuse and manipulation, and choose to behave nicely with you. The next chapter discusses these aspects in detail.

Chapter 5: Set Healthy Boundaries, Become Assertive And Don't Give In To Unacceptable Whims And Irrational Behavior

One major reason why narcissists continue to overpower you is because you allow them to by not establishing healthy boundaries in your relationships.

Boundaries are crucial to success because they help the people involved in a relationship understand the parameters of the bond and what they must and must not do.

For instance, if you do not ever talk to your friend about how you do not appreciate the fact that he/she lies to his/her mother about spending time with you whereas he/she is actually hanging out with his/her drug addict friends, he/she is likely to continue with that and throw more dirt on you.

Similarly, if you don't tell your narcissistic spouse that his/ her dominating behavior annoys you and that he/ she must sort out their act if he/ she wants to continue living with you peacefully, he/ she will only continue to do the same.

Chances are that your spouse may still behave the same way even if you communicate your concerns with them, but if you keep acting decisively, you will be able to modify their behavior soon.

Here is what you need to do to become assertive with the narcissists in your life and change their irrational behavior.

Understand What You Want and Set Boundaries Accordingly

First and most importantly, spend some time reflecting on what you expect from your relationship with the narcissist. Wrap your head around one thing: he/ she is incapable of loving you like you hope for, and while there is hope for them to improve, do not expect them to transform into a completely optimistic, supportive and loving individual because their thought process has now become quite distorted.

So while thinking of the expectations you have about them and how you would like for them to behave with you, think as rationally as possible.

List down the things you want that person to keep in mind when interacting with you and set boundaries accordingly. If you want your partner to stop playing the blame game, communicate that concern with him/her. If you want your sibling to stop yelling at you every time you don't pay follow his/her demands, inform him/her of that firmly.

Make Sure the Boundaries are respected and Reach a Compromise with them

When you do set certain boundaries with your narcissist partner or friend, make sure he/ she observes them. Keep a check on his/ her behavior and if you observe him/ her breaching the limits, have a firm talk with him/ her one last time. Even if you do not wish to leave him/ her, tell him/ her that you may have to do that if they push you to that and in that case, separate from him/ her for a few days if the need arises.

Also, inform the narcissist that you are only living with them or carrying on with the relationship you have with him/ her if they choose to compromise. Talk to them about how suffocated you feel and how you are now in the position to live independently, but since you have spent quite a long time with them and respect that, you wish to stay on good terms with them if they respect you back. Be very firm when you say that and try not to cry or show your emotions because that again can weaken you and put them in the power position.

Play with their Feelings like They Do with Yours

Always remember that a narcissist in any relationship views the other person as his/ her competitor. There is no concept of having the middle way in a relationship or giving love, as they expect to receive because they only expect to get what they want irrespective of their behavior with the other person.

In any relationship, they can only see in terms of the top dog who is like the alpha dog, giving directions to others and an underdog, one who pays heed to the top dog and tries to act more like him. A narcissist only wishes to be perceived as the top dog, so when you try to turn things around, he/ she is likely to become hyper-alert and look for ways to return to the alpha position.

They have quite an inflated ego which they do not want to lose at any cost. So when you try to act assertively with them, they will play even harder to hurt you and will always act as if they are competing with you. So if you try to hold your partner's hand, he/she may jerk yours to hurt your feelings. If you ask your friend to go out for drinks with you, he/she may refuse your offer to cause you pain.

If you wish to outsmart a narcissist, you need to go as low as possible to match their emotional frequency. You can do two things. First, you can give him/ her regular assurance that you are not competing with them or trying to prove that you are better than him/ her. This should be in case that narcissist is the vulnerable type. If he/ she belongs to the grandiose category, you too need to hurt him/ her a little. Stop making attempts to appease him/ her when he/ she is upset; do not go out of the way to make him/ her feel comfortable; and stop checking up on him/ her to ensure they are doing okay.

Just look after yourself and do not act as his/ her guardian or care taker at all. When you stop tending to his/ her petty needs and acting like his/ her care provider, he/ she will soon realize that you have changed. He/ she will then try to hurt you or apologize to you. In both cases, inform him/ her of how unacceptable his/ her behavior is and that you will not take any of that nonsense again. Remember to be firm at all costs and you will only break him/ her further.

Use the Word 'NO' when Needed

Throughout our lives, we have been told that 'sorry', 'please' and 'thank you' are the 3 magic words you need to use to win people's hearts. While this is true, these words often do not work with narcissists. In fact, they only give them too much reassurance which makes them get on your nerves.

To effectively and tactfully handle a narcissist, you need to create a new vocabulary of magic words for him/ her and the first word in the list is 'no.' Narcissists yearn to hear 'yes' to everything they demand from others. If they want you to stand on one leg the entire day, they expect you to oblige. They want you to take them on expensive trips and they won't hear 'no' for an answer. Often, the problem in narcissistic relationships is that due to the fear of upsetting a narcissist, you are likely to say 'yes' to all his/ her demands. While you hope for your sacrifices to make him/ her a nicer person, he/ she won't ever change.

Instead of agreeing to everything he/ she wants, start saying 'no' more often. If a narcissist comes up with an unacceptable demand, firmly reject it. Yes, it will upset him/ her and may even make him/ her act irrationally, but you need to stick to the 'no' in any case. Just do it a few times, distance yourself from them and do not budge from your stance in any case, and within a couple of weeks, they will get used to hearing no from you. While they may stay grumpy, so be it because you need some peace as well.

Challenge them

Narcissists lie in different and strange ways. Sometimes, they exaggerate things to come off as a superior individual, and on other occasions, they can fabricate the biggest of lies to bring you down, or even make fantasies involving them. This can be very annoying and if you keep up with this behavior, you will only play a role in inflating their ego.

You need to challenge them by asking them for a proof every time they make a claim that seems false. Demand evidence that proves their claim and clearly show that you doubt their story. When they feel challenged, they are likely to budge from their stance, or stop making stories the next time.

Tell Them They Don't Scare You

A good way to neutralize someone with a narcissistic personality is to inform them of how they do not scare you. Such people are insecure and wish to turn on the insecurities of others too. They observe the insecurities and weaknesses of others to exploit them when the need arises.

If any narcissist you would like to change does that to you, fend him/ her off by telling him/ her of how his/ her tactics do not scare you. If he/ she becomes furious, let him/ her explode because that is clearly not your problem. Do not comfort him/ her at that point because again, that is not your concern.

Don't Talk to Them Until Necessary

Do not talk to your narcissistic friends or loved ones unless absolutely necessary. When you try to neutralize their effect, they will want to get back to you.

So your partner told you she is upset and needs you, but you know she only wants to try her hand at controlling you again so you tell her you are busy. This is likely to challenge something which will compel her to try to talk to you time and again. When that happens, avoid talking to her completely.

You need to prove to the other person that you are strong enough to survive on your own, and can do really well in life even when they are not around. Since narcissists are lonely and do not have many people to seek support from, when they see you drifting apart, they are likely to improve on their act.

If you do see the narcissists in your life improving after a few months, show them compassion and love, but always in moderation because too much comfort can again put them in the power position. Soon, the two of you will establish a workable relationship that will neither burden you nor him/ her. However, if he/ she becomes abusive to the extent that he/ she resorts to physical, sexual and extreme psychological abuse to manipulate you, it is best to think things through and bring in a lawyer and legal authorities to save yourself from any irreparable harm. While you may not want to leave him/ her, there may come a time when you have to, and in that case, it is best to save yourself now than feel sorry later.

Conclusion

We have come to the end of the book. Thank you for reading and congratulations for reading until the end.

This book holds within its parameters great power, but only you get to decide how to use that power. The ball is in your court; use the information wisely and get started with improving your life now.

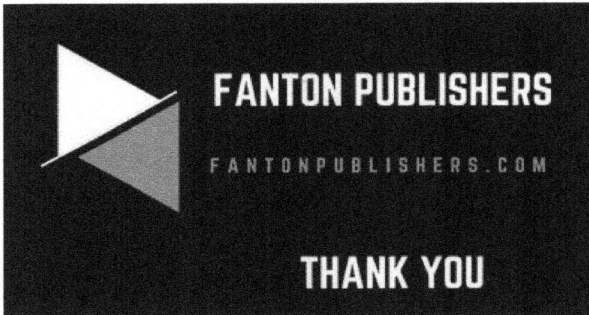

Do You Like My Book & Approach To Publishing?

If you like my writing and style and would love the ease of learning literally everything you can get your hands on from Fantonpublishers.com, I'd really need you to do me either of the following favors.

1: First, I'd Love It If You Leave a Review of This Book on Amazon.

2: Check Out My Emotional Mastery Books

Note: This list may not represent all my Keto diet books. You can check the full list by visiting my author page.

[Body Language: Master Body Language: A Practical Guide to Understanding Nonverbal Communication and Improving Your Relationships](#)

[Shame and Guilt: Overcoming Shame and Guilt: Step By Step Guide On How to Overcome Shame and Guilt for Good](#)

[Anger Management: A Simple Guide on How to Deal with Anger](#)

Get updates when we publish any book that will help you master your emotions: http://bit.ly/2fantonpubpersonaldevl

To get a list of all my other books, please fantonwriters.com, my author central or let me send you the list by requesting them below: http://bit.ly/2fantonpubnewbooks

3: Grab Some Freebies On Your Way Out; Giving Is Receiving, Right?

I gave you a complimentary book at the start of the book. If you are still interested, grab it here.

[5 Pillar Life Transformation Checklist](#): http://bit.ly/2fantonfreebie

www.ingramcontent.com/pod-product-compliance
Lightning Source LLC
Chambersburg PA
CBHW031135020426
42333CB00012B/386